Rachel Lafferty lives in a small town on the north coast of Northern Ireland. She lives with her partner and young son. She enjoys nothing more than a big cup of coffee and a book. Rachel has written *Pandemic in Paradise* during lockdown 2020.

For my son, your mummy's doing her best. I'll love you forever. For my partner, I might not always say it, but I appreciate everything you do for me and our family. For my aunt, I hope you're looking down on me, this book is dedicated to you. You never got to meet my son. I love you, and I miss you every day. I hope that I'll make you all very proud of me.

Rachel Lafferty

PANDEMIC IN PARADISE

AUSTIN MACAULEY PUBLISHERS™

LONDON • CAMBRIDGE • NEW YORK • SHARJAH

A CIP catalogue record for this title is available from the British Library.

ISBN 9781398464988 (Paperback)
ISBN 9781398464995 (ePub e-book)

www.austinmacauley.com

First Published 2024
Austin Macauley Publishers Ltd®
1 Canada Square
Canary Wharf
London
E14 5AA

I would like to thank my family, partner and son.

2020 was the year of COVID-19 coronavirus. This deadly virus which took the entire world by storm, and ultimately shut our entire country down amongst other countries around the globe. The year when I was pregnant and gave birth to my first child. The year when it was difficult, heart-retching, complicated and very fucking messy. This is my personal story of being pregnant and being a new mummy throughout a global pandemic in the UK. This is to the endless days spent indoors, clapping for the NHS on our door steps, not being able to get a Tesco delivery slot, overwhelming statistics which led to countless deaths, hopes and fears for the future and for our children and families. No schooling, lack of education, no income leading to poverty, working from home and days of self-isolation leading to depression and self-deprivation. Unprecedented times. Probably the most used term of 2020 used by the UK government and leaders around the world.

It all began in early January 2020 when I attended a doula course in Belfast, Northern Ireland; something I was highly interested in. I love learning and I'm always interested in the more quirky and different approaches to studying and life. My brain goes at a hundred miles an hour, I always need to be doing something, anything to keep myself busy and out of mischief. I'd briefly studied psychology at The Open

University, among other things, at secondary school when I was younger, but this really grabbed me. I was excited about meeting my group and becoming a professional doula, and of course helping women throughout the entire childbirth experience. Childbirth is probably one of the most important but traumatic experiences of a woman's life. Women were travelling from all over the UK to meet in Belfast. My home city.

Whilst there, I became ill with what I thought was a stomach bug, I couldn't eat much and was constantly on the toilet, shitting my guts out. I remember running around boots looking for Pepto-Bismol, anything to help soothe my tummy for thirty minutes. My tutor, who I grew very close to and would regard as a close friend, knew straight away even before I did what was wrong with me. I spent all day sipping on the stuff like it was vodka and coke.

For some unknown reason, I thought I could be pregnant; my period was around a week late, but for me that wasn't unusual as my cycle was always very irregular. I had a strange feeling that I needed to buy a test, just to rule out being a parent right now. I wasn't exactly ready to be a mother. Me and my partner hadn't exactly been safe, so there was always going to be a chance. I wasn't one for contraception of any sort, I was almost against it, because my hormones were already so fucked up, I didn't want them to be even more so. I'd never ever been on anything, not even the morning-after pill.

I went out to the shops and purchased two pregnancy tests just to make sure. It's one of those things I've always felt really embarrassed about. I don't know why… I always felt like the lady or man behind the till in the pharmacy were already judging my impending motherhood. I wonder if they thought to themselves, "Oh Lord, this wee girl is in for a hell of a ride if she's pregnant" or "Bless; good luck to her" or maybe just felt really fucking sorry for me. "Poor sod." Taking the test and finding out I was pregnant wasn't a shock, but a realisation that my life was going to completely change. I wasn't going to be able to do the things I had done before; I certainly wasn't going to be able to travel the world anymore. I wouldn't have any time for myself, I wouldn't be able to just lounge about all day and read countless books and binge watch the tele. Me and my partner would have zero time together. It was certainly going to be a process, trying to readjust to a new way of living with a new human being.

It's one of those things; I was actually craving to have a baby, any which way possible; my body just wanted to be pregnant. It's something I kept thinking about in the months leading up to finding out I was pregnant. My maternal mothering instinct must have kicked in, and I just knew that I was already producing a little human being. A mini me. Or more like a mini version of his father. A shitting, eating machine.

Growing a life inside you is the weirdest and strangest feeling ever, the body is truly extraordinary. Those first little kicks, that well, you aren't sure entirely if they are kicks or possibly what you ate for dinner the night before, repeating on you. Due to this wide-spread pandemic, maternity services had gone completely tits up. Partners weren't allowed in with the women at all, even at scans or their antenatal appointments, nursing staff were rushed and pushed to their limits. Therefore, they didn't have much time to spend talking to the women, or offering any kind of useful advice or support, bar leaflets and printed sheets of well cow shite, that is common sense, and if you don't already know those things then maybe you shouldn't be having a child right now.

I was already truly scared about what it's going to be like giving birth. "Am I going to be completely alone…?" "What happens if something goes wrong, and I have no one to comfort me?" "What if I die?" "Is anyone going to know I'm dead?" "What about the baby?" "What size is he going to be?" "What if he gets stuck in that canal thing?" My mind had gone into full on fucking overdrive. I basically had to live in hope that everything was going to work out in the end.

The older nursing staff I found are so bloody rude and not living in the 21st century, which was already giving me huge anxiety. From the get-go of my pregnancy, I've found them extremely patronising. They just really pissed me off. They're just not up-to-date in anything that goes on in the modern world today; they've got their old school ways of doing things, and God help you if you question that. You're the worst person in the world to question their authority and how they do things.

"What if these old bitches are the only ones with me whilst I'm going through the worst pain in my entire life?" Harsh as it may sound, but it's the truth. I honestly hoped and prayed they wouldn't or someone was going to get some choice words from me. You need someone who's supportive and doesn't question what you want; after all, it's MY baby and as the old saying goes, "Mum always knows best".

Having children hasn't really ever been something I'd put much thought into when I was younger, I mean I knew I only wanted one child but whether I'd birth the child myself, I was never entirely sure of. But when I met my partner, I felt happy and comfortable that the relationship was stable enough and I'd be happy to have his child. We both met online, which is what all the youth of today do, nobody just meets on the street or in a pub anymore. I went on there to find someone; I didn't actually think I'd find the father of my child! Let alone the love of my life! We took the risk, and met in Cardiff, Wales, his home city. Once we met, that was it, we were smitten. We both wanted the same things in life; children, nice things and to be our own wee family unit. We've both struggled growing up, having various problems and obstacles to overcome. We've both struggled with depression and mental health problems, and know what it's like to be hurt, and hung out to dry. We have a lot in common which is always good, and we just really clicked and understood each other.

He wasn't in a great situation back in Wales, and I was chuffed that I could help him out, and hopefully give him a better life with me. He's lived in Northern Ireland now for around three and a half years, although he'll admit it's not his favourite place, as it's very religion heavy. He's here for me and the little man, not all the drama and other shit that goes along with living in a political society full of bullshit. Someday, we are planning to move elsewhere, but for the meantime we're as comfortable as we can be, where we are. A nice big new house for Christmas would be great, so big man if you're really up there, give me a break and answer my prayers, eh? Possibly throw a wad of cash my way too! Amen!!!

Fostering a child/children has also always been something I've thought about. I didn't have a very good childhood myself, and I always thought about trying to give a child who's maybe not had the best start in life, a better chance, a clean slate. I'd always read these books as I got older by a lady that I really looked up to. I can't mention any names, but she's such an inspiration to me.

She's fostered hundreds of children throughout her life with a partner, then on her own when her marriage had broken down. She just kept going on helping more and more children. Maybe in the future or something, I'll look into it more. I'm highly aware that most children in the care system have been through a lot of trauma in their young lives. I'd never want my own biological child or children to suffer because of that. I don't care what anyone says, but you will always have more of a connection with your biological child, which again is concerning because you've got to try and love them all the same, and nurture them as if they are biologically your own child. In some way, you've got to be the parents or have careers that they never ever had. You've got to give them that unconditional love they never had or ever felt.

A key aspect of having a baby is making sure you are 1. In a healthy relationship or environment and 2. Being financially stable and having a loving home. A lot of people I know don't have this and it's sad, everyone deserves happiness and love. A baby is hard work, and having now a nearly four-month-old, it's really bloody tough work. It takes over your entire life and your personal routine is out the window. Plus, it's even harder being in lockdown and not being able to take my son anywhere, or get him involved in any wee groups. As babies get older, it does indeed get easier.

I remember when my son was first born, he needed to be fed and nursed every four hours, so even if he was asleep, we would have to wake him, to make sure he didn't miss a feed, then it took so long to get him settled again and back to sleep again. As he grows, he's becoming so much more independent and will be able to play and feed himself soon enough. Which gives me time to scratch my arse.

His routine now is better. Thank the lord, I couldn't cope if he stayed a new-born forever. My mental sanity would be long gone. At least he's become a little more self-sufficient. He seems to only wake once for a bottle at night, which is OK I guess but if he wasn't such a greedy little mite, maybe he'd sleep the whole night through. He definitely takes his huge appetite from his father. He loves his food and will scream the house down and get himself into a right state if he doesn't get it in zero point two seconds.

I'm a little fussier, I'm a small and regular kind of gal. Coffee is my muse. I need caffeine on tap every morning without fail. It's not pretty until I've had my morning caffeine fix, then I can deal with whatever hell is thrown my way.

I was always scared to have my own child as I didn't have a great childhood myself. I made the decision when I found out I was pregnant to start going to therapy again. Proper therapy, not the leaflets and forms the GP makes you fill out to determine how depressed you are, then make you scale it from one to bloody 10, just to see if you're depressed enough to receive the help. I've always had a lot of demons to fight throughout my life, they seem to follow me everywhere I go. I just can't shake them off. I first started going to CAMHS (Child Adolescent Mental Health Services) when I was 17. I felt like I needed to improve my wellbeing and be the very best version of myself for my child and of course myself at 26 years old. It's been a long process and it's still an ongoing battle. I was truly terrified of my parents' parenting rubbing off on me, I didn't want to be anything like them at all, so for me I needed to work through those issues to better myself. I honestly couldn't live with myself if I had turned out anything like them.

I've got to constantly remind myself each day that I am my own person. I'd been so detached from myself my entire life; freezing they call it, because you've gone through so much trauma, your body just freezes up and doesn't let you have any kind of emotional response. Because your body wants to protect you in any which way possible from any pain or suffering.

I'm still going to therapy to this day. I've got a great therapist, I wish I had found her years ago and if I'm honest, I probably will be in some kind of therapy for the rest of my life. My childhood was so damaged that it damaged me as an adult. I haven't fully found my identity yet, and that's OK. I'm still figuring life out. It's only been since I hit my late teens that I realised what I had gone through as a child shouldn't have happened. I've always said, I would never be on any anti-depressants if it weren't for my parents.

Enough about me, back to cute little babies. It's the most amazing little life you'll ever get to know and produce. Babies are born utterly resilient and thrive on love and attention. There was very little help from anyone throughout my pregnancy. I had to basically research everything I wanted to know. I'd spend hours reading articles about feeding and sleeping. I didn't get much support from any nursing staff or health visitors either; I was completely isolated without anyone. I'm lucky I had my partner, but even so he wasn't allowed in with me to appointments or scans which was very frustrating and upsetting. The first time I properly saw my baby, I was alone for my 20-week anatomy and gender scan.

Of course, I would have loved to share it with him but even so it was still magical and a true bonding moment between me and my son, which I also think is important for my mental stability. I remember seeing the penis and I was like, "Well, it's a boy then," and she confirmed it right there and then. For some reason, I thought I'd always have a girl, but it really didn't matter to me. As long as the baby was healthy and well, that's all that really mattered at the end of the day.

The 20-week scan is the big one. At the scan, not only can you find out the sex of your baby, but also if there are any complications or serious medical problems. I cannot begin to think of what it must have been like for women who were totally alone to be told that something is wrong with their baby or worse, that maybe their baby wouldn't survive the pregnancy. I can't even comprehend what that must have been like for them.

A lot of women were also denied to take any kind of pictures or videos of their child to show their partner and family because it's against hospital policy. Looking back now, there should have been something more in place for this. Not only are you affecting the mother's mental health by denying her this but you're also upsetting the partners and family and denying them a chance at seeing the unborn child. It was an awful situation, and I feel like it shouldn't have happened in the way that it did. The prospect of going through an, interesting to call it, entire pregnancy alone without my partner was very daunting and scary. Not only was it my first pregnancy but there was a global fucking pandemic.

Because I'd never given birth before, I didn't have a clue what to expect, let alone what it would feel like. I mean, I know it certainly wasn't going to be pleasant from what I had learned in child development at high school. Looking back now, all the videos you watch or books that are out there never fully prepare you for it. I remember asking women what it was like and reading articles about birthing experiences, and it did not describe or sum it up at all. I also think women who've had children don't want to actually tell first-time mums how bad it actually is, because if they did, the poor souls would be terrified.

I would be brutally honest; it's bloody terrible, and the pain is off the bloody scale. My advice, take all the drugs they offer, it won't take the pain away but it does help! Women are now expected to go through most of the birthing experience alone, due to COVID-19 restrictions and regulations; birthing partners are now not allowed into the room with the woman until she is in active labour (4–6cm) dilated.

I spent a full night in hospital before I was finally induced the next morning. My son was then born the following day and 24 hours after I gave birth, I was then discharged home. I was so ill when I was discharged that my partner and my dad had to carry me upstairs in my home, because I couldn't walk after the spinal block injections. I shouldn't have been discharged so early because I then went on to spend two weeks upstairs in my house because I couldn't walk back down the stairs. When I did eventually get to sleep, I'd wake up in tears, crying that I was in so much pain, because by then the all the pain medication I was given had completely worn off. I also went on to have multiple infections which were treated with five or more courses of antibiotics. I felt like after I gave birth, I was rushed out of hospital so quickly without any tools, help or support. They'd even forgotten to do my son's hearing test, which is always done in a hospital setting once an infant is born, so we had to travel 30 miles to another hospital a few weeks after he was born to get it done.

I didn't have a clue what to do with my baby when I got home. It made me very depressed and I'd feel so much guilt for not being able to look after him properly. It's very heart-breaking for fathers because they are also made to leave pretty much straight away once their baby is born. Men don't get the test for coronavirus before the woman is admitted, so I don't know if this is the reason behind not letting them stay? It must make fathers feel pretty useless, the mum has gone through the most traumatic and painful experience of her life then is left alone, with a new baby.

When I was on the ward alone at night with my son, I'd just stare at him and wonder, *What the fuck do I do next!? What do I actually do!? Nobody has told me what to do!?*

My experience is my own thoughts and feelings on giving birth during a global pandemic, the way I was treated is not to say that every other woman out there is going to be treated the same. I did not have the best experience during my labour but I also think it's because I wasn't given the tools or advice to help me through it, because there was no help available due to the coronavirus outbreak. The birthing experience was very traumatic and when I think about it now, it still makes me feel very emotional and very let down by the National Health Service. I know we're in a truly awful and devastating situation, but it affected maternity services really badly, to the point where pregnant women's care wasn't at the standards it should have been, and we women suffered because of it. I don't know if this would have happened if COVID-19 hadn't been around, but if it wasn't here and I was treated the exact same way, I definitely would have made some complaints about my care. But if I could afford private treatment, I would certainly have paid for it.

Saying that, I've recently learnt that a lot of private health care during the pandemic were actually giving their beds to the NHS because there was nowhere for COVID-19 patients to go. The NHS were already under a huge amount of pressure in 2020 when the first wave hit. My first-born baby boy was due in September 2020.

My symptoms throughout my pregnancy weren't all that bad, compared to some horror stories I had read on Reddit; it was the tiredness and the morning sickness which mainly hit me damn hard. I started having morning sickness at around 17 weeks, which to some women is quite late; normally, morning sickness occurs at the early stages of pregnancy. It got to the stage where I'd get up around 8am and be back in bed by mid-day. The pain I experienced in my spine during pregnancy, especially in the third trimester, was extremely painful, due to the condition I have in my back where my discs are fused together. Therefore, I cannot stretch my back straight. With the weight of the baby and fluids which was probably around half a stone by then, it was getting utterly exhausting.

I slept all day and all night, I slept like a big fat bellied Buddha. I hadn't gained much weight at this stage, so I was starting to be concerned about how big my baby actually was. I've quite a small frame so I wasn't expecting to gain stones, but I know it is healthy to gain some extra pounds during pregnancy. Each time I'd go for a scan, it was always a different consultant, and because they were always so busy and normally only one member of staff on, I'd also have to sit and wait for two hours before I was even seen. When they'd measure the baby, they'd either say "he's perfect", "great size" or they'd say "he's too small". So, to be honest I didn't know if he was going to be OK until he was born which caused me great anxiety throughout the end of my pregnancy. I was constantly on edge that something bad was going to happen to him. Thank the lord he was born at 6 pounds 14 ounces at 41 weeks and 6 days on the 3rd of October 2020. He was a well-cooked bun in the oven.

Of course, I would have loved it if he had been born naturally, I tried holding off on all medical intervention as long as I could. I was offered a sweep on multiple occasions, but I declined, to try and give my son more time.

Unfortunately, he was just far too cosy, snuggled up in my womb, using my bladder as his pillow. Also babies that spend longer time in the womb are scientifically proven to be better off and more developed and even smarter. Little Einstein I've got.

So, let's go back to January 2020 when I found out I was pregnant. Fuck! My next step was to obviously confirm my pregnancy with my doctor. Once the doctor confirmed I was pregnant, it was like it's really real now. First advice I was given was to start iron supplements and to stop my antidepressants completely, cold turkey.

That was the completely wrong advice as two months later, I was begging my GP to put me back on them again. Although, when you're pregnant, it's just not as simple as the doctor prescribing them again, no, you've got to see a mental health professional to determine whether you can or not. So, the medication that I'd finally found that worked for me, that I'd been on for around a year, someone told me to stop, even though they shouldn't have, they weren't going to give me them again just because now I was pregnant. I fought tooth and nail to get my medication back again. I did eventually; but I was given a lower dose which amazingly I'm still on; 60mg lower than I was on before to this day. It is a small victory, because once he arrived, I was told I'd have to go back to my original higher dosage. My mood has stabilised a lot since I've given birth, it's my fucking time of the month that really fucks with me. I'm going to have a baby. A little human being who is going to be totally reliable on me. Who will need everything from me for the next 18 years of their life!

After our first scan, nurses would start the whole breastfeeding talk. "You should really breastfeed!", "It's better for your baby!", "You should stop your medication and do it!", "DO IT NOW!" Firstly, I was on meds my whole life; antidepressants, heart medication and pain relief. They are something that I NEED for my health and wellbeing. I couldn't just stop at a click of a finger; the withdrawal wouldn't do me or the baby any good.

Taking medication during pregnancy has always been controversial. In my opinion if you really need it, take it. I was so calm throughout my pregnancy, I don't know if that would have been the same story if they hadn't let me stay on my medications. There is just not enough scientific evidence to prove that it will in any way harm your unborn baby, especially in regards to antidepressants. I'd spend sleepless nights dreaming of this deformed monster baby after what the doctors would tell me, that scare-mongered me into thinking I was going to be doing so much harm to my unborn child. I thought I'd end up killing him. I was advised multiple times to stop taking my medication, but I made the correct decision for me and my baby. He was, of course, born perfectly fine and healthy. It just goes to show that YOU always know your own body and what is right for it. There is nobody that knows you better than yourself. Of course, there is certain medications that you cannot take during pregnancy, but for me I made the choice which suited me and my body.

The start of my pregnancy was very stressful. We moved from a relatively nice rented home to an extremely rough council estate. I found this extremely difficult because in my mind I'd let my son down already. The estate itself wasn't in the middle of the town, but the outskirts. There was litter, beer cans and dog shite all over the pavements. The house itself had boarded up windows and no central heating. It was an absolute fucking disaster. We're still in the estate to this day. Due to COVID-19 restrictions, it's proving harder to get a privately rented home, because obviously nobody wants to move in the middle of a global pandemic. It really affected me mentally and really brought me down.

I wanted everything to be perfect for him, a beautiful home garden etc, and this was the exact opposite. All I wanted was a nice, comfortable home for me and my family. The house was a complete shit heap, it was disgraceful. There was zero heating, so much so that the pipes had actually been removed, dog shit throughout the home, and around 20-plus repairs that need to be done. We did manage to get some work done before the baby arrived but to this day, everything has not been done.

The "housing folk", shall we call them for legal reasons, in Northern Ireland are the people who rent social housing out to those in need or those who find themselves homeless, and I can honestly say they do not care about their tenants. They probably go home to their beautiful homes with their beautiful partner, plush rugs and quality food. I bet they haven't ordered a munchie box for one to share between two.

They are money grabbers. When I'd kick off about the house and the way it was given to us, they'd use every excuse in the book to get out of it. It was always someone else's fault! I felt like the biggest failure on the planet. We weren't in the most ideal situation for this baby to be born, but we had a roof over our heads, a warm home (eventually) and we had enough money in the bank and food in the cupboards. We were looking forward to welcoming our little bundle of joy. The most upsetting thing that I had to try and get my head around was my family not being able to properly meet the little man. You weren't allowed to mix households, so I couldn't take him to meet his great grandparents, who are extremely frail, and my biggest fear was anything happening to them before they'd even get the chance to meet him. The most important thing a baby needs is unconditional love and lots of cuddles. A child will love you unconditionally because as a parent, you are fulfilling their wants and needs.

Life has definitely changed since I've had my little one; time with your partner of any romantic sort has completely vanished! When you have a baby, you and your partner ultimately become a team for life, regardless whether the relationship lasts the length of time or not. You've got this one little person that you've got to raise for 18 years, they've got to be guided into life, to then live their life on their own. It's probably one of the most important jobs in the world.

My parents didn't know what to do with me growing up, my childhood wasn't the best. My parents separated when I was one year old, they never spoke ever again. It was always weekend drop offs and pickups. It was like a rivalry, what one could outdo the other, which one could always do better. Pick a side, heads or tails. In hindsight, looking back as an adult, what I went through as a child, at the hands of my mother, was pure neglect and abuse. Obviously, as a child you don't know what's right or what's wrong, you trust your parents, you always believe that they must be right.

I was very depressed as a child; I remember first being depressed when I was seven years old. I'd cry myself to sleep for no reason, I was just really fucking sad. It terrifies me that I might not be the best parent I can be to my son, and because of my childhood and my parents, I'm very hard on myself. I never give myself a break or a pat on the back.

Let's go back, I seem to be rambling on… my son was born a healthy 6 pounds and 14 ounces at 41 weeks and 6 days. I was taken into hospital the day before I was due to be induced, and was finally induced the next morning.

My partner basically had to force the midwives to let me have a bed. I was told to phone every morning from 40 weeks to get a bed. Every morning, there was none. The risk gets higher the further along you go, the placenta can stop working, and then the body doesn't produce all the vitamins and minerals that the baby needs.

Giving birth was definitely the most painful experience of my life, and I can say I really don't want to go through it again. I made a point of writing in my pregnancy notes and birthing plan to not under any circumstances be in any way patronising. I couldn't think of anything more annoying than someone saying "well done" "good girl" "great job" whilst giving birth, I am not your pet and you're not puppy training me. Although I wouldn't entirely rule out having more children, but probably not birthed by me and my very extremely weak and tired body.

As long as I've remembered, I've always had physical and mental health problems. I was born at 32 weeks weighing like 3 pounds and the size of my father's hand. I was extremely ill and due to that I got a narrowed blood vessel to the brain (stenosis) and a disease in my spine (kyphosis), as well as a heart problem (SVT). I didn't learn about these health concerns until I was in my early twenties, when I started to get ill. So, in general when I get any illness or sickness, I get it twice as bad as a healthy person. It hasn't held me back, but I sometimes struggle to do everything that I want to.

Time is the main problem when you decide to have a baby; there's never enough hours in the day to get the things done that YOU want to. I'm quite a creative person, so there is always a project I want to work on. I normally try to rush everything just so I feel better about myself, like I've actually achieved something for myself in the day, other than cleaning shit off the surfaces. I've always struggled with mental health problems, like depression, disordered eating, anxiety and OCD. So, most of the time the things I want to get done, I don't necessarily need to do. Little rituals to make my soul happy. I'm still trying to find the balance between being a mummy, a partner and well just me.

For as long as I remember, I've always been different and I've always known that something just isn't 100 percent with me. That my brain works differently from everyone else. That I see and feel the world different from everyone else. But I've never been able to just put my finger on what it is. After I gave birth to my son, I underwent lots of tests, and found out I had multiple strokes as a child, which was never picked up on, which is no surprise. I was so neglected as a child that my parents never noticed anything about me. They never saw me. When I was seventeen, I was diagnosed with Anorexia Nervosa and my parents did absolutely nothing. They sat back and watched their daughter waste away and basically slowly kill herself.

I proceeded to try and take my own life, which may I add they didn't notice and then I left home at seventeen, once I'd discharged myself from hospital after downing the activated charcoal to rid my system of the cocktail I had ingested, with no clue or idea of what I was going to do or where life would take me. I just got up and left and to this day leaving, getting out, being free, it's the best choice I've ever made.

Sickness and nausea is something I've also suffered with; I've always got something going on. And because I was born premature, I tend to get sick more than other people. I try my best to look after myself but getting the time these days is very difficult with a four-month-old. He needs constant attention and care. It's a very demanding role, being a parent is probably one of the most important roles you can play in your life. It's basically like being a full-time carer; you've got to feed them, clean their arse, wash and bathe them. Your child doesn't need everything, your child just needs you. Your baby only knows you and your soul. My son loves to sleep on my chest, babies love the sound of their mother's heart beats, it reminds them of being in the womb. All cosy and wrapped up, unconditionally in love with you as you are with them.

My health throughout pregnancy was relatively good. My mental wellbeing was fucking amazing. Throughout my pregnancy, I was probably in the best mental state that I've ever been in, in my entire life. I felt like I was untouchable, a real force to be reckoned with, a pregnant superhero (if one exists). Although, because I've suffered with mental health problems quite badly in the past, they automatically put you in the "this mummy needs a closer eye on her" group. They'd make me see a psychiatric nurse at every anti-natal appointment, without even asking me if it was OK or if I agreed to seeing someone, which I fucking hated. I would get rants from the midwifes about suicide rates and how I should consider their therapy. "Sorry, love, I've been there and done that, stitched, sowed and made the t-shirts myself." I made multiple complaints to the trust that I did not need any help. As appreciative as I was that this kind of help was in place, I'd rather the support go to someone who really actually needs it and wants to receive it.

Now that I'm out of pregnancy and I've fully recovered from the birthing process "#4 trimester", my hormones are now up the shitter. Thankfully, I've got a very calm, understandable and patient partner. He deserves a gold medal because I'm an absolute hot mess. My hormones are a nightmare to say the least. Two weeks before my period, they start playing up. Then when bloody Mary finally decides to make an unwanted appearance weeks later, thanks to my irregular fucked up cycle, I turn into a raging psychopath. On the hunt for chocolate, arguments and sweet treats.

Children are an unknown species, in the sense that you never know what they bloody want, what they need or how they feel. "Hungry?" "Sleepy?" "Need a poo?" "Want a cuddle?" "What do you want? Please tell me!" Babies until a certain age cannot express what their wants or needs are. That's why it's so difficult when they're so small; you almost have to try everything over and over again until something works. "Change the bum", "try the bottle", "read the book", "throw the ball", "dance around the room, jump up and down or just lose the fucking will to live".

My son is definitely the light in my life (cliche). He's so funny, a proper wee joker, such a troublemaker. If we as parents raise him correctly, he should grow up being "kind", "generous", "compassionate" and "always kind towards others". These to me are the key components of being a well-formed fully functioning human being. If he's more than that, that's amazing and we'll know we've done the job well.

Nobody is a perfect parent. Maybe online you can see people that are looking like it, but the truth is you're going to mess up and get things wrong. If any parent is out there who's never put a foot wrong, you're either a miracle worker or a fucking good liar. It's all about trial and error, especially if you're new to the world of being a mummy or a daddy.

People who have more than one child, I take my hat off to you, you are amazing, force to be reckoned with, I don't know how you do it. When do you sleep, eat, have a shit? Some days, I don't even have time to change my knickers or wipe my arse. Maybe I only say that because I have one and the lack of sleep has put me off anymore. God, I miss my bed. It's those small things you miss once you have had a baby; uninterrupted coffee, watching a series on Netflix, reading a book or just having a bath without constantly hearing a baby crying and screaming in your head. It's like having tinnitus, of constant screaming and crying. I remember going to bed one night, and the baby was with his dad in the other room. And I woke up in a panic thinking I'd taken the baby to bed. That's fucked up!

New parents always get advice thrown at them from every

direction, some of it not welcomed might I add. When I was pregnant, I was basically told by midwives I MUST breastfeed, it wasn't even suggesting that maybe I should. When I said no, they'd say "Oh so you can't be bothered then?"

"No, I take medication, so no, I can't." Which again I'd be questioned about why I wasn't stopping the medication. It's a game of cat and mouse, me being the tiny mouse trying to get the fuck away from them. I will do what I think is best for me, myself and I. Not everything is about the baby. Yes, the child is important and will consume your entire life but I'm still here too. I still have my needs. If I don't look after me and make the decisions that are best for me to look after him, then I'm not going to be well enough to be his mummy.

Being a mummy is tough, and I don't want to sound in any way sexist but it always seems to be portrayed in the media that the fathers are always absent. My partner is probably one of the most hands-on dads out there; he loves doing everything with our son and always jumps to the occasion of taking him from me. Dads get a bad name and image. When I came out of hospital, my partner did everything for me and my son because I was so poorly. I couldn't lift my baby, feed or change him. When the time came and I felt like I could, I had to ask my partner "So how do you change a nappy?" "How do I feed him?" "Am I doing it correctly?" Because we had no antenatal courses or classes, we both didn't have a clue. Looking at it now, five months on, it's like riding a bike, it feels so natural. Human instinct kicks in and you know you've got to care and nurture this small human being, who is so vulnerable and can't do things for themselves.

Pregnancy throughout the COVID-19 crisis has definitely been challenging. Parenting has also been tough; no mummy and baby classes or schooling available. Everything has been remote and from home. This I think has definitely affected young people's mental health and especially their educational needs.

I wonder whether this will damage my son's learning and skills when he's older, because I haven't been able to take him out as much. He hasn't had the chance to interact with other children his age. I would have loved to be able to take him to a class, have him physically play and learn with other children. It's almost like COVID-19 has robbed him of his first important months in the world. It's lonely, sometimes depressing, especially when my son was first born. I didn't know what to do, I wanted to take him out for a walk but was terrified of people coming up to the pram, scared stiff that he would catch this virus. It also took me two weeks to be able to look after him when he was born due to complications in my labour, so I felt pretty shit. That when he was most vulnerable, and I couldn't help him, I couldn't be the mummy he deserved. I still carry a lot of guilt about that.

I had my labour all planned out, of course plans can change, but I wasn't expecting to not be able to do anything for my son. When the contractions finally started after I was induced, they were mild to begin with, quite manageable with gas and air. I was given a birthing ball, and was just bouncing up and down like the Easter bunny. But as they grew stronger, the pain at the bottom of my spine just became far too strong. I couldn't make my mind up whether I wanted an epidural, because I knew that it came with complications and side effects. It also wasn't fully part of my plan. I wanted as little medical intervention as possible. I actually wrote that I wanted a water birth in my birthing plan. I tried the water, but it seemed to make the pain even worse. So I decided to just do what made me feel better. I knew that if I got any kind of spinal injection, I wouldn't be able to walk or move about. I'd be bed-bound completely. I was always told by the community midwives that the less medical intervention you need, the easier it is.

In the end, I decided to take the epidural; the consultant came in and attempted multiple times, but due to the condition in my spine and the fused discs, they couldn't get the catheter into the space it needed to go into. My partner hates blood and could well pass out at any minute, so I was angrily shouting at him to leave the room. The last thing I needed was for him to be in the bed next to me. I was desperate. Every time I was having a contraction, they'd have to stop putting the needle in. I'd shout "CONTRACTION!" and they'd pause and wait for it to pass.

They eventually had to call in another consultant specialist who had to do a spinal block, which is only normally done in surgical settings for women having a C-section. When he had done it, he said, "Oh some fluid is coming out" and I was like "What wait! What do you mean!? Am I going to die!? What is happening!?" I went into full panic mode, I kept asking the midwife who'd been with me from the start if I were going to die and she wasn't really giving me the answers or reassurance I needed. I just wanted everyone in the room to tell me I was OK. I craved that. I was sitting there bent over, with a huge needle in my back and there was fluid coming out. That to me didn't sound promising.

They did eventually say I was fine, but for that brief period of time, I thought I was going to die. Usually when this happens, and fluid is leaking, it normally means it's coming from the brain. I was in utter panic, totally terrified that I wouldn't be able to make it through this labour. It was all getting too much. I just couldn't cope anymore.

Unfortunately, the main issue with the spinal block is that it wears off super quickly, in around an hour; so it constantly needs to be topped up with the drugs by the anaesthetist. So, every hour on the hour, they'd have to call down the specialist from the intensive care ward to top it up and make me more comfortable. It definitely took the edge off the pain, but the pain was so strong it was still really unbearable. Then all of a sudden, out of nowhere, I really needed to push. I'll never forget that feeling, I was screaming, "I NEED TO PUSH", "PLEASE SOMEONE HELP ME, WHY AREN'T YOU HELPING ME?"

The only way I can explain it is as if you need a really, really, really huge shit, and you need to get to the toilet and go, or you're going to explode and shit is going to be flying everywhere; it's so intense. It's fucking awful. I feel like everyone romanticism giving birth, as if it's this beautiful experience, orgasmic even. NEVER doing it again, and never putting myself or my body through it again.

The midwife who was managing my care had gone on her lunch break and they wouldn't let me push until she arrived back, because it was some trainee nurse and I don't think she had a clue what she was meant to be doing there. I didn't care who did what, I just needed this baby out of me NOW. It was the most extreme pain I've ever felt or gone through in my life. She rushed back from lunch, she looked and checked me over and was shocked that I'd jumped from 4cm to 10cm and was ready to push. They put the hand railings up and my feet basically touched the ceiling in the air.

I screamed and screamed; they kept telling me to be quiet but I didn't care. If you've ever watched one born every minute, and you see the woman losing their fucking shit, screaming like primal animals, it's a verily accurate representation of what I was like. Then the baby just slid out, just like a baby otter emerging from the waters; sorry, been watching too much of David Attenborough in lockdown. He was placed on my chest, not crying but safe and well. He looked all around the room, at the people, the lights and his surroundings. He was so alert. It was amazing. I was so emotional; I was in tears, I kept saying how beautiful he was. It was like a real-life fairy tale, with the most beautiful ending.

I'm needlessly in love with my son, he just brightens up my day. Anytime I'm in a really shitty mood, I just need to look at him or give him a big cuddle and I instantly feel so much better. When parents say that they couldn't imagine life without their children, it's a billion percent true. They give you such a purpose in life. A reason to keep going and get out of bed in the morning; well, not as if you're going to be getting any sleep for the next 18 years of your life, but then the worry probably won't disappear.

A lot of women after pregnancy really hate their body, their stretch marks, scars, the unwanted cellulite, fat and the weight gain, of course. I've always seen magazines with celebs always trying to shift "that annoying baby weight" to get the most amazing post-pregnancy bod. I actually didn't really have to worry about that. Around two weeks postpartum, I had lost all the baby weight and nearly half a stone of my pre-pregnancy weight. As nice as it was to have my body back to some kind of normality, I knew the rapid weight loss wasn't normal nor healthy, I shouldn't have lost so much weight so quickly.

I kept taking quite sharp pains in my abdomen, and these continued for months after pregnancy. Sometimes, they're called after pains, when the womb contracts down to its size before pregnancy, but this pain wasn't right, it didn't feel normal. It was progressively getting worse by the day.

I paid to go see a private doctor. Once I'd seen him, from there, I got a lot of scans and tests done to try and determine why I can't gain weight anymore. To this day, I'm still waiting for results back and for the doctor to figure out the underlying issue. My weight seems to be stable at the moment but I'm nowhere near my pre-pregnancy weight.

The one thing I hated after pregnancy is definitely how saggy my skin has become, especially my under arms. I feel like I'm ready to take flight at any stage with my bingo wings. *Caw, caw, caw, caw,* here I come! My partner of course keeps reassuring me that it's because I haven't worked out properly in a long time, and since I'd been sitting on my arse for nine months, that obviously my body wouldn't be strong or tight!

On the topic of things being tight, my vagina will NEVER be the same EVER again. I leak all the fucking time. So much so that I'll probably be wearing the same nappies as my son for the rest of my life. Ladies, please do your pelvic floor exercises like the midwives keep telling you. I didn't and well, I'm sitting here like a leaky faucet now, or a garden sprinkler that's on a timer, you never know when it will go off.

Now I'm five months postpartum, I'm doing everything and loving it. Sometimes I overdo it but he's worth it. I think all mothers can say that they'd do anything for their children, it's a primal maternal instant. To protect your own, like the mother lion protecting her cubs, she would never let any harm come to them, she would die for them. I'd do exactly the same for my son.

Looking back now on the first lockdown, it was a really tough time, I spent my entire pregnancy from January 2020 until October 2020 indoors. I think I must have read 50 plus novels. Reading is one of my past times, I spent hours in bed, with some chocolates and a coffee. My god, what I would give to be able to do that now. It was just me and my partner, my family lived in another town and because of the coronavirus weren't allowed to travel unnecessarily. My partner's family all live in England and Wales, so there was no way we'd been able to see them. He has a fairly good relationship with them, so we know they are always there if we need them.

I went out possibly once a month to go shopping but spent the rest of the time shielding. When I hit around 30 weeks, I stopped going out completely, there were a couple of reasons behind this: 1. I was terrified I was going to give birth early, quite literally in the supermarket. 2. I couldn't walk that far because I was so big. I spent so much time indoors, so much so that it would start to take its toll on me. You find after being indoors for a few weeks that you start to get cabin fever and all you can think about is getting out of the house and being anywhere but stuck in your living room. You honestly feel like you're going to start climbing the walls, it makes you go a wee bit loopy. It feels like a never-ending story. It's all you see any time you switch on the television, it's taken over our lives. Its ruined lives, taken lives.

COVID-19 is a right bitch and a horrible one at that. It

has no compassion for its victims, it doesn't care about loss or grief. I still honestly cannot believe sitting here today that we're still in the midst of a global pandemic, something I didn't even think was possible in this lifetime, let alone in this century. I had my son in a global pandemic, it's definitely going to be some story to tell him when he's older. It still amazes me that even in this lifetime we'd be struck with a deadly virus, and that there was no way of stopping it from spreading, no vaccines available until a cure could be made and mass testing was conducted.

I'm lucky enough that I have in fact received my first dose of the Pfizer-BioNTech vaccine. Due to my work in a care home with dementia patients, who are extremely clinically vulnerable, I was offered the vaccine. Part of me felt extremely guilty for taking it, as people who are seriously ill and elderly hadn't even received it before I had. I remember asking the nurse if I could give my vaccine to my grandmother who has dementia herself and she said unfortunately it doesn't work like that. I'm 26 years old and although I do have underlying health problems and would eventually be offered the vaccine, I'm well off compared to some people, and very lucky. There was initially a tier system of who would get the vaccines first, I would have been at the bottom of the list if it wasn't for my voluntary work in the care system. I feel truly blessed for that, because I'm protecting my family now to some extent.

"How long would this virus be around?" "How long would it take us to make and produce the vaccines on a global scale?" "When would we be able to get the vaccines?" "When will our lives go back to normal?" "Will there ever be a normal again?" These were just some of the questions that everyone was asking. We are all desperate for those answers. We are all desperate for some normality back into our day-to-day lives. A routine. Obviously, there are idiots out there who are anti-mask-wearers and anti-vaccine this and that. Those people are the reason why we cannot have our lives back.

I remember going out for a walk with my partner along the river, pushing my baby son in his pram, having a big massive cup of coffee and saying, "Do you know what I miss the most?"

"What?"

"Just fucking breathing, just breathing in air."

Wearing masks indoors all the time is so frustrating, annoying and extremely suffocating. I wear glasses, and it's like entering the ghost train every time you go into M&S; I can't see what I'm buying. I don't have the foggiest. (Very punny)

Now it's 2021 and again, still stuck in the rut of being indoors with a now five-month-old isn't easy. I have nowhere to take him, I can only take him out for a walk, and even at that I put a plastic covering over him in shops or in situations where there are a lot of people, because I'm terrified of people touching him or getting too close. The furthest we get now is either out to the backyard, a walk or to the local shop.

The virus is hopefully showing signs of slowing down, deaths seem to be far reduced than they were but we're still not safe. Gone are the days of just being able to fill your lungs with fresh air. Gone are the days of going out for a spontaneous coffee or catching up with your mates. My anxiety surrounding going out gets too much sometimes, but my son is getting to the age where he's getting more and more curious and wants to see and explore the big world outdoors.

I can't keep him under lock and key forever. I try to make things as interesting as possible for him, but sometimes, he settles and relaxes better being in the fresh air and hearing the little birds chipping and different sounds in general. I just want him to have a normal childhood, like everyone else has. He's already missed out on so much at the early stages of his life.

"Is this going to become the new normal?" "Will it just be normal to wear masks as he grows up?" "Will it be normal to self-isolate?"

I just want the world to be the way it was before coronavirus threw a spanner in the works. We will all get through this. Together. One day at a time. It will get easier. The end is approaching. I hope for all our sakes and sanity.

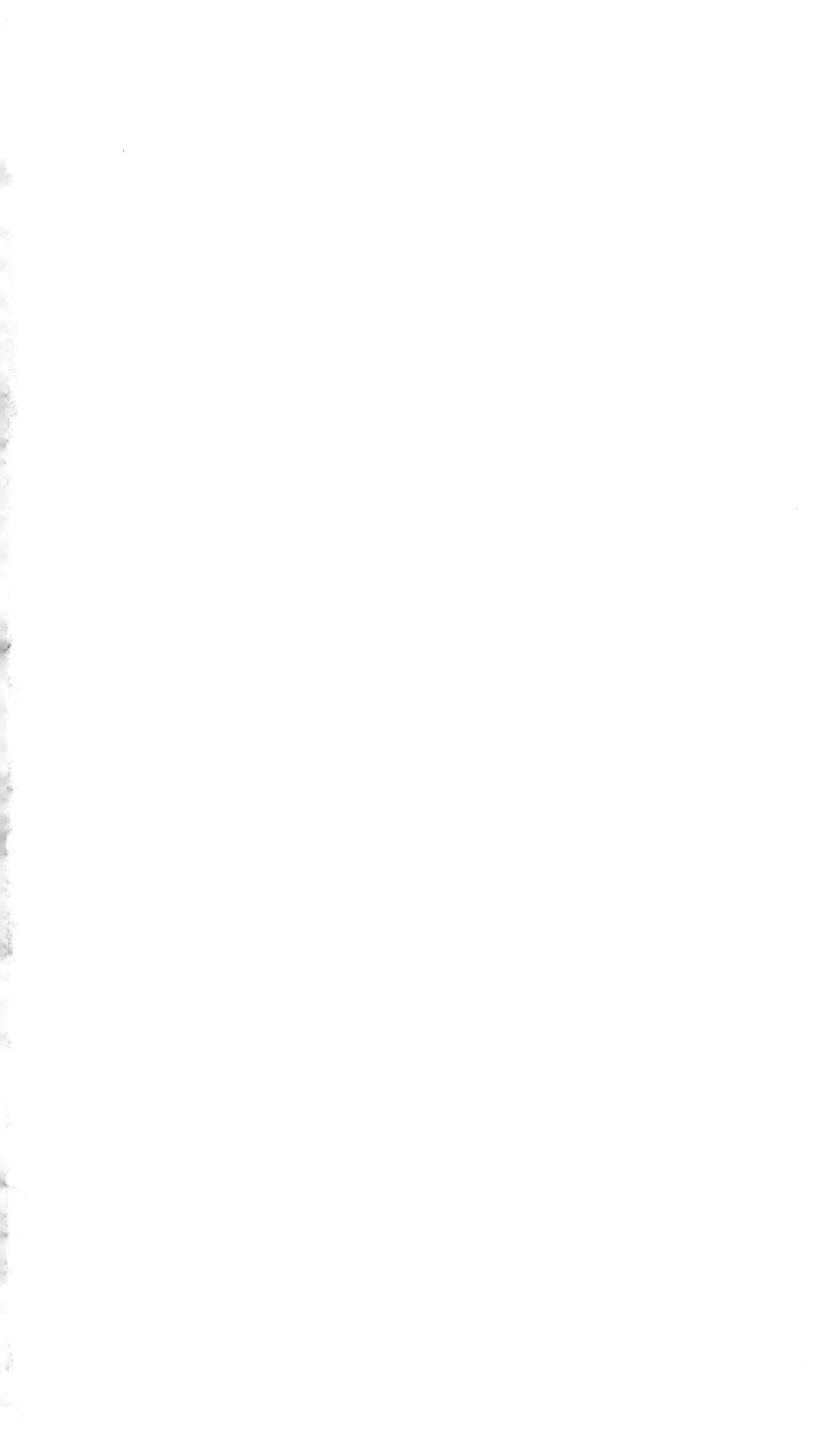